Special Things To Do During 3 Hours of Sex: A Step-by-step Guide

Copyright (C) 2013 by Phil G.

ISBN-13: 978-1481092708
ISBN-10: 1481092707

Erotic BDSM Books - Your Erotic BDSM Book Publisher
EroticBDSMbooks.com

This publication includes two free bonus books (making it an $20.85 total value!) Your books are presented in this order:

BDSM Books by Phil G. Include:

BDSM Master/slave Contract
The Absolutely Essential Book of BDSM and S&M Rules
Things To Do During 3 Hours of Sex; A Step-by-step Guide
Playtime At The Dom Den; A Step-by-step Guide
The Absolutely Essential Guide to Great BDSM and S&M Sex
The Absolutely Essential Dominant/submissive Playtime Experience
The Absolutely Essential BDSM Sexual Experience
The Ultimate Collection of S&M and BDSM Rules For Female Submissives and Slaves
Master and submissive or slave BDSM Contract
Have Awesome BDSM Sex
Spanking Dictionary
Spanking Contract
BDSM Rules
Bed Arrest, the Punishment for BDSM Enthusiasts

Book #1
Special Things To Do During 3 Hours of Sex: A Step-by-step Guide

Just a quick bit of information about my lovemaking style, I am a sexually dominant, heterosexual. I need my lady love to be able to orgasm-on-demand, or agree to be trained for it. Typically she's trained to have extremely long orgasms versus several comparatively shorter ones. This is part of where my sexual dominance comes in. My lover will need to start her orgasm quickly, and continue it for as long as I am sexually stimulating her by using my hands or other parts of my body. Fortunately the human female body is built to have long, frequent and powerful orgasms, though so comparatively few women get to enjoy their incredible built-in capacity for pleasure. The truth is that orgasm-on-demand is a remarkably easy thing for women to do once properly trained.

Most men concentrate on a woman's body to stimulate her sexually, (which in and of itself is not a bad idea) but in so many cases that's not enough. I have found that most men do not adequately sexually stimulate their women's minds.

There is a natural tendency by women to be the more submissive sex during sexual activity, and that would certainly be required for the 3 hour playtime we're discussing. (Please note that if this tendency toward submissive behavior is not true in your case then this type of orgasm on demand training likely won't work too well with you.)

In her now sexually aroused state, it's normal for her subconscious mind to be more susceptible to suggestions regarding sex. People like me take it a step further and require her to do more than that during her sexual submission, specifically she will be required to orgasm long and hard, no ifs, ands or butts. Thus it is no longer her decision on how hard and long to orgasm but her lover's and I for one will require her to orgasm relentlessly.

Another way to look at it is that after being trained for orgasm on demand, the woman no longer is the one making the decision as to when *she* is going to have her orgasms and/or how intense the orgasm will be. She has yielded that responsibility to her lover and her mind fully accepts his/her authority in the matter.

Let's remember, a woman's subconscious mind doesn't usually care who tells it to begin orgasming, it can be her own mind giving the order or it can be her lover's. As a woman you just have to be in the right frame of mind to let it happen.

For 3 hours of sex it is very helpful if the man lasts a long time and/or is capable of getting hard frequently and with minimal downtime.

I last an extremely long time, usually for at least the whole 3 hours. I also have a thick penis which of course is a help.

Incidentally if someone is looking for an easy to find penis desensitizer cream, over the counter hemorrhoid cream under the tip of the penis can work well. I would urge the man to test it out on himself before being with a woman as if too much is used he might not even feel the stimulation enough to get hard! The man needs to know just the right amount to use and chances are it's a small amount.

I wanted to note that the dominant sexual position discussed in this book works best when the woman is no more than somewhat overweight.

Here are specifics of what we'd do in our 3 (or more) hour playtime.

1. When you enter my (our) place, you will take off your shoes and go kneel on the thick padding next to my bed (or other agreed upon spot like a chair or couch). Unless told otherwise, your eyes will be looking at where my midsection would be when I sit down in front of you. You will wait for me there (unless of course I'm already there.)

2. I will come over and sit in front of you (assuming I'm not already there.) I may or may not have clothes on. You'll then put your hands on my upper legs, massaging my legs with anticipation. Keep your hands high up on my legs, massaging my legs but you may not touch my penis until allowed to.

3. I will kiss you, touch you, play with you, talk to you and undress you as you kneel submissively in front of me. At some

point you may be ordered to stand up and take the rest of your clothes off. Unless you're told differently, in private, as a slave you should feel uncomfortable with clothes hiding your private parts from your Master. They exist for his pleasure after all!

4. You will partially or fully undress me when I order you to. When you pull my pants and underwear down, you know what will pop out!

5. I will then let you suck on my penis. You will first likely have to beg for it though. Also, remember to always play with Master's testicles while you suck...always!

Rule: Never let any of Master's penis' ooze go to waste. You know good it tastes! Beg Master to let you check for ooze often! Keep sucking Master's ooze down until he allows you to stop.

6. Soon I will reach down and play with your exposed, vulnerable breasts as you suck on my penis.

7. At some point I may order you to stop sucking my penis. If so I will tie your hands securely together.

8. I may order you to suck on my penis again or we will go straight to the following:

I will sit further back on the bed (or couch/chair) and you will lay stomach down across my lap. I will give you a nice sensual spanking, playing with your body as I do.

I will then tell you to get up and we will go to the bed (if we're not already there.) I will set the bed up so I am sitting with my back against the headboard of the bed and you are laying in front of me face-down on cushions with your head positioned so you can easily suck on my penis and play with my scrotum using your tied-together hands. If I do that though I will make sure there is enough slack in the rope for your hands to still move freely around my penis and scrotum while you suck. If your hands are tied to the middle of the headboard in this manner, I will be sitting on the rope as my butt will be in-between your bound hands and the headboard which your hands are tied to.

9. I'll also put a roughly 4' x 3' (though it can be larger) sheet of plastic under your upper body to keep the massage lotion or oil from going on the bed covers. (More on this massage very soon!)

Your breasts will now be positioned, thanks to cushions, so the bottom tips (which will likely be the nipples) of the breasts are just above the bed. As you are lying down and sucking on my penis, I will **generously** lubricate (and keep lubricated,) your breasts with some brand of preferably non-desensitizing lotion or massage oil. (I prefer lotion. Baby lotions at dollar stores often are good ones to try but lotions can vary by brand.) The longer the lotion can stay viscous, the better. If warming is necessary (which it most likely will be,) I will warm the lotion/oil up ahead of time or rub it in my hands to warm it up. I will then massage your breasts as you suck on my penis and play with my testicles.

I will continue for a long time to massage your lubricated breasts as you suck on my penis. (This is known as *"Extreme Pleasure Breast Massage"*.) **Remember massagers, <u>always</u> keep you're your hands well lubricated!**

Massager and massagee will quickly notice that the nipples respond with the most pleasure from this type of massage. The Dom will find that massaging his slave's breast's large fleshy area first for a while will be quite pleasurable to his slave but it is still not near as pleasurable as briskly massaging her nipples with a circular twisting motion that lets the fingers slide firmly over the nipple, not actually twisting it.

I will first make my slave beg to have her nipples massaged using this *Extreme Pleasure Breast Massage* technique. My slave has no more than 30 seconds to start her orgasm when I first start giving her *Extreme Pleasure Breast Massage.* Once I start massaging her nipples, she will have to orgasm a lot harder or risk being punished.

Using a yardstick type implement, I can also reach across your back and spank your bottom as you suck. Obviously one should make sure the woman can handle being spanked while sucking. Most can depending on the intensity of the spanking and how hard she's already orgasming.

Optional: After doing this for some time, you may wish for the lovely lady to be turned over on her back, her hands still tied to the bed. The man can then eat her. The lady should plan on providing her Master or Mistress a lot of pussy juice. Should she not provide you with enough pussy juice, feel free to turn her over so her bottom is facing up, and give her a good spanking. Then try eating her again. (Before playing it is important that the lady keep her pussy clean and fresh.) After you've had your fill of her pussy juice, both of you can go back to the original position mentioned in this section or move on to #10.

10. At some point, I may also tie each foot to its corresponding corner of the bed. Instead I may tie your feet securely together and then tie them to the middle of the bed frame at the foot of the bed. Don't worry guys, the placement of a woman's vagina on her body while she's laying on her stomach is such that you still most likely will have easy access even with her legs closed. (This could be a problem depending on how overweight she and/or he is.)

11. At some point I will order you to stop sucking by saying "head up". I will then get up and give you another spanking as you lay tied down, just for good measure. If you've been a good girl and are getting a lot of pleasure from all this, *and if you beg for it,* I will put a special vibrator (or two) inside and/or on you and set it up so it stays in place. (Tight underwear and white first aid fabric tape often works best where there are pubic hairs in the area.) I will then return to my original position on the bed and you will continue sucking me and I will also continue giving you *Extreme Pleasure Breast Massage* (which I promise you'll enjoy immensely!) I will continue to periodically spank you with a yardstick type implement as described earlier.

12. After a while, I will order you to stop sucking. I'll then clean the lotion off your breasts with a small towel(s) and remove the small plastic sheet that caught lotion that came off your breasts and my hands. I'll also remove the cushions from under you that kept your breasts just above the bed. You are now comfortably laying face down on the bed but now without the cushions and plastic under you. You still however are tied down to the bed as you lie on your stomach. (You may wish to put a clean towel under her breasts if they are still a bit oily from the massage.) I will remove any vibrators on and/or in you, as well as whatever was holding them in place. You will be completely naked, tied down, helpless and ready to be taken.

13. I will come back in front of you and order you to suck on my penis again. After it is hard, I will dry it off and put a condom on it. I will then lay on top of you, stomach down, and enter you with my thick penis.

14. As I take you, you will orgasm for as long as I order you to and orgasm as hard as I order you to. You are required, as part of the orgasm on demand training, to start orgasming within 5 seconds of me entering you. Believe me it is much easier than it may sound. You will need to ask for permission to start orgasming though! As long as you start asking for permission within 5 seconds of me entering you, you are doing fine. Of course you will need permission to stop your orgasm also! There is the possibility that at some point I will order you to stop your orgasm during our lengthy playtime (or obviously you may have to do that due to unexpected events like the kids coming home early.) If you can however, you are welcome to keep orgasming even though direct sexual stimulation has temporarily stopped; (for instances after I have stopped taking you.) Once direct sexual stimulation of your breasts and your vagina restarts, you'll of course have to re-start your orgasm once again (assuming it had stopped,) and within 5 seconds as always. (Many of the ladies I have trained will continue orgasming for many minutes after physical sexual stimulation has stopped.)

15. As I take you, you will orgasm for as long as I order you to and orgasm as hard as I order you to. Believe me young lady, I require long, hard orgasms from you.

16. As you know I am taking you while both of us are on our stomachs. My stomach of course is on your back. This is far and away the main position I will take you in for the entire time I take you. I may also take you doggie style depending on how overweight the slave is. There will however not be an emphasis on multiple sex positions during our playtime.

RULE: while I'm playing with you, if you are lying on your stomach and if I ever say "elbows" you are to raise your chest enough so that the tips of your lovely breasts are just above the bed, thus making it easier for me to play with your breasts by sliding one or more of my hands under your chest as I am taking you.

(I think you'll find that *my stomach on your back position* to be a very good one. Depending on how heavy and/or tall the guy is, you won't have any trouble breathing as my weight is well distributed over your bone-protected pelvis. You won't have to deal with my breathing on your face or you being pounded against the headboard like in the missionary position. Also I can hold you tightly as I take you and easily talk to you as my mouth can be right by your ear.

17. At some point I will slide one or both of my arms under your underarm(s) and put my hands on or around your hands. I am now securely holding you down with my hands. You can now reach my hands (as they are on your wrist, forearms or hands) and kiss them should that be our desire.

RULE: while we are playing you will only address me as "Sir" or "Master".

18. Sometimes while I am taking you like this, I will spank you. This is accomplished best by me holding myself up with one

hand/arm while I am in you and then spanking you with a paddle or the like with the other hand.

19. Often I will hold you down while I take you. I will order you to struggle *FROM THE WAIST UP* to get free as I am holding you down and taking you at the same time. We will do this one or more times during our long playtime.

20. Sometimes I will take you faster than other times. You will get even more pleasure from this as most any woman would.

21. Sometimes I will thrust into you as deep and hard as I can. You will get even more pleasure from this as most any woman would.

22. This is an excellent sex position for a lady to be taken anally. Perhaps she should have her anus lubed in the beginning when she is originally laid in place incase her Master/Mistress decides to take her anally.

RULE: *Remember, the man must always wear a condom when taking her anally and he **can not** re-enter her vagina unless his pubic area has been thoroughly cleaned. A bladder infection is just one of the problems she can have if one doesn't abide by this essential safety tip.*

Remember, if something is hurting young lady, you need to tell your Master immediately so he can stop.

Well so there are the sexy details of how to play for 3 (or more) hours! Have fun!

The End

BDSM Books by Phil G. Include:

*BDSM Master/slave Contract
*The Absolutely Essential Book of BDSM and S&M Rules
*Things To Do During 3 Hours of Sex; A Step-by-step Guide
*Playtime At The Dom Den; A Step-by-step Guide
*The Absolutely Essential Guide to Great BDSM and S&M Sex
*The Absolutely Essential Dominant/submissive Playtime Experience
*The Absolutely Essential BDSM Sexual Experience
*The Ultimate Collection of S&M and BDSM Rules For Female Submissives and Slaves
*Master and submissive or slave BDSM Contract
*Have Awesome BDSM Sex
*Spanking Dictionary
*Spanking Contract
*BDSM Rules
*Bed Arrest, the Punishment for BDSM Enthusiasts

This book is sold and/or distributed with the understanding that the publisher and author is not engaged in rendering legal or other professional services. **This book and its subject matter is for entertainment purposes only.** In this publication there may be inadvertent inaccuracies including technical inaccuracies, typographical inaccuracies and other possible inaccuracies. **The writer and publisher of this publication expressly disclaim all liability for the use or interpretation by anybody of information contained in this publication.** The author, publisher and distributors of this publication hereby disclaim any and all liability for any loss or damage caused by errors or omissions resulted from negligence, accident, or any other causes. If legal advice or other expert assistance is required, the services of a competent professional person in a consultation capacity should be sought. Products, services and websites' content vary with time. Please verify any published information.

Copyright © 2013 by Phil G.

Book #2 - Entertaining Kinky Personal Ads

Entertaining Kinky Personal Ads

Introduction

This book provides entertaining excerpts, and complete kinky personal ads, from sources throughout the world. The emphasis is humor and other forms of entertainment.

There are numerous volumes and this is only volume one. Be sure to read the other volumes too!

There is a lot of information online as to what BDSM is. This book however is not written in an effort to advocate it. This book likely is not one of the better reference sources regarding kinky exploits as it's oriented to humor and often highlights the absurd.

The content of this book is a lot like bathroom graffiti humor and a good deal of it is not particularly respectable. Just a warning ☺

As these terms come up often in the book, let's make sure you know what they were:

Dom - Short for the *Dominant* person in the relationship.
Sub - Short for the *submissive* person in the relationship.
Slave - The submissive person in the relationship.
Master - A male who usually is the controlling person in the relationship.
Mistress - A female who usually is the controlling person in the relationship.
Domme, FemDom, FemDomme - A Mistress, a strong woman in the relationship.
Collar - A symbol of the submissive belonging to the dominant.
Vanilla - The normal non-bdsm respectable world.

Between each "¤" in the book is a new personal ad or excerpt that is unrelated to the personal ad or excerpt above it or below. *(This will make more sense after you start reading the ads.)*

Table of Contents

Dominant Women Personal Ads & Excerpts

I am everything you have ever wished for in a Domme. I am strict, yet loving; bitchy, and still sweet. I may punish you until you cry, but I'll be there to caress you and help you understand why it had to be that way. I am seductive, sensual, bitchy and snotty all wrapped up in one exquisitely beautiful package. You're a lucky boy if you can get My attention and keep it.

¤

You're a worthless maggot, a waste of life, a pathetic little fucker who doesn't deserve anything more than dumpster diving for food in order to keep me happy. You are a weak, sad little man who needs the control of a strong Goddess to put you where you belong: groveling at my feet.

¤

No one else will understand a lost soul like you the way I will. I know all about those sick thoughts that are running around in that pin sized brain of yours. So treat yourself to a session with me.

¤

STOP HERE slaveboy! Mistress is ready to be worshiped, adored and served! I will love training you and doing what I wish with you. I will punish you slowly and make you beg for mercy. Come here and kiss My feet and lick My boots like the slave you are!

You will beg me to allow you to touch yourself, you will beg me to allow you to look at me! I am your new owner now! I own your mind, your body and soul! I take you wherever I want from you! You are my property!

¤

All your fantasies will become real with Me, because I am not only a great looking Mistress with sexy body and hypnotic eyes, but I also know how to get I want!

¤

Domme window shopping for a new sub.

¤

You are just a slut, a whore to your needs and willing to do whatever it takes to grovel and beg for release. Be comforted in the knowledge that your Mistress has heard this all before ... and there is very little you could say that hasn`t been pleaded for before.

¤

I'm looking for a sub girls to play with, use and abuse. I'll fuck you with my girlbreaking strap-on. Our sessions will be long, hard and fun! You will serve me with forced orgasms and anal. Everything and anything is available for me to use on, and with you...

¤

Mistress looking for pain pigs, male or female.

¤

I am an open-minded, sadistic, 28 year old dominatrix. I am now actively seeking worthy submissives to serve Me both online, in real-time and financially.

¤

I'm looking to meet a slave to use as my property. I want to own your heart, body and soul. I'll enjoy having you...

¤

You will build your Mistress a dungeon.

¤

This is your Mistress speaking, don't just dream about crawling into captivity under the cruel and capricious control of the superior sex, DO IT.

¤

Life's a bitch, so am I.

¤

I decide who may or may not be my pet. I decide who may participate in my filthy fantasies. You won't get what you want, but I will...and if you don't do what I order, you will be thoroughly punished.

Submissive Women Personal Ads & Excerpts

I have been into BDSM for just over a year. I've met some great people and one jerk.

¤

Submissive female looking to explore BDSM. I particularly enjoy playing a school girl or patient. My real school girl outfit from 8 years ago still fits.

¤

I like books, movies, music, walks in the park, being tied up...

¤

I like to be tied up and gagged but I'm not into anything serious.

¤

I am a petite sub girl that likes to misbehave...and get what comes with it!

¤

Only the one that hurts you can make you feel better.

¤

I definitely enjoy being submissive to a partner both in the bedroom, and to some extent outside of it, but I am far from perfect in this, so if told to do something I don't want to, I will generally try to negotiate my way out of it at first, but ultimately accept that I am not the one in control and obey. And the masochism? Oh how I love a good beating. Beat me until I scream and cry and beg for mercy and I will be calm and happy for days.

¤

Come'n'get me if u dare. Turn offs: bad breath, poor personal hygiene and the inability to finish a sentenc...............

¤

Each month my Master makes me a list of goals to be completed within a certain time period. One of this month's goals is to have a sexual encounter with another female. I've never done this before, so I am looking for someone that will take the lead. Master wants me to be a more well-rounded person and this is an area that we decided needed to be addressed.

¤

I have sub tendencies that rear up from time to time and at those times I find myself on this site more than I should be. At other times I happily retreat into a vanilla haze. I don't know what it all means but for now I have needs.

¤

I need someone to show me the ropes!

¤

I am a very sexy pervert.

¤

I swing both ways in most things I do.

¤

Interested in life, love, happiness and water sports.

¤

Bi female, naturally submissive, 5'4", blond hair, needs a spanking.

¤

I like being controlled, I love feeling powerless - that squirmy adrenaline rush when I realize I no longer have a choice. I will be absolutely devoted to someone who makes me feel uncertain, jumpy and eager to please. I will search for their touch, and bend myself into shapes in order to get them to notice me.

¤

I've worn a chastity belt and they itch.

¤

Pain is just pain to me, (though sensation play is wonderful!) If I wanted to endure agony, I'd have kept my last job working in insurance.

¤

Lost girl looking for her Daddy. I'm willing to do as Daddy says and want to please him and make him proud of me.

¤

I love to be tied and teased. I need to be used as a sex slave. I am witty, friendly and deliciously horny.

¤

I want to be a slave, a plaything. I want to be used and abused as Mistress sees fit and to be punished as warranted. I want to be collared and milked when needed.

¤

I've been told that I need a spanking.

¤

Somebody signed me up to this site. She only just told me about it. Wow, the things people wrote saying they wanted to do to me. You should be ashamed of yourselves.

¤

Sub bitch that needs taming.

¤

36c and into most kinks and perversions.

Dominant Men Personal Ads & Excerpts

Looking for intelligent lady who needs instruction.

¤

I'm seeking a bad woman for good times. I'm ready to let loose the hell fires of lust.

¤

I'm a love technician and I have lots of rope.

¤

If you're a grown up school girl, a naughty wife, a bratty daughter or just a very kinky young lady who needs more discipline in her life, you should message me immediately! I can be whoever you'd like and take all your troubles away. I can also provide lectures and motivation to help you reach and maintain your goals, and let's not forget about the spankings.

¤

My sub died, I need a new one.

¤

Forced homosexuality, Nipple torture, Corporal Punishment, Medical Scenes, Rubber dolls, Spitting, Toilet play, Humiliation, Adult Baby play, Dehumanization, Needle play, Electrics, Pony play, Piercing, Anal play, CBT, Boot worship, Verbal abuse, Waxing, Bondage, Degradation, Ashtray play, Full latex enclosure, Financial Slavery, Objectification, it's all there for us to enjoy.

¤

Homicidal maniac seeking victims.

¤

Dominance in the Hood!

¤

Bound for Topeka?

¤

I'm a tongue fucker. Sit on my face young lady and feed me...When you're done, it will be my turn.

¤

Dominant male seeks obedient slave girl with dripping pussy and nice tits that wants to be used as sextoy.

¤

Interested in meeting like minded folks and leaving teeth marks all over them.

¤

Mature male, very experienced, seeks schoolroom games including role-play; age-play; interrogation; ritual discipline and restraint.

¤

I'm looking for a willing sub to learn from me. Submit and we will find our true path.

¤

I'm happy to introduce newbies. I have expertise in corporal punishment, bondage and orgasm control. I will test your boundaries. I am demanding but fun.

¤

Show me that smile.

¤

Mean, cruel dominant male. Write me now!

¤

I'm getting more sadistic as I get older.

¤

I'm easily annoyed at girls who just can't behave.

¤

Ladies if you're into cock worship, you're going to love Mr. Mike.

¤

Viking looking for a maiden to capture.

¤

I love aggressive cunts.

¤

It's fun corrupting the nice girls and punishing the bad ones.

¤

My perfect woman enjoys endless nights of restraint and teasing.

¤

Looking for some slaves to play with and perhaps even become partners in crime.

¤

I am an experienced Dom who can be VERY strict but also very caring. I'm looking to expand my learning with a willing student. I'm usually heterosexual.

¤

Live-in and all facilities provided. The lucky slut who catches my eye will be a masochist, exhibitionist and fun-loving. The qualities that I find most pleasing are honesty, obedience and compliance. If you fit the bill, are prepared to become my property, and are looking for a good home, then email me and we'll have a chat.

Submissive Men Personal Ads & Excerpts

I'm a empathic clairvoyant. I'm a visionary and my perception of others is more like a spirit guide directing souls to find their true inner beauty. I'm a spiritual entity who practices a karmic flow. I follow a born calling and work as a shamanic healer, clairvoyant and directional counselor. I like hallucinogenic drugs and days without bathing.

¤

My name is Bob and I have balls.

¤

There's nothing like being choked while being wanked.

¤

I'm not into emotional blackmail (but sexual blackmail is fine, in fact encouraged :)

¤

No pain no gain.

¤

All I really can say is lgg kfkflkn fflafsng fgasgsfasf sdfaffrfr.

¤

I'm here to exchange perverted thoughts and look at naked breasts.

¤

I believe in tough love.

¤

Mouth gagged, hands and legs tied to the bed, then comes a long spanking. Your fantasy or mine?

¤

Old man looking for new tricks.

¤

Submissive male with smoking fetish. Into bondage and forced smoking.

¤

Can you handle a man like me, I doubt it.

¤

I'm a kind, cultured, intelligent gentleman who likes to wear dresses.

¤

I am willing to submit to real punishment including spanking/paddling if you decide that I warrant it. I would rather have a sore butt than an unhappy girlfriend and going over a woman's knee certainly leaves no doubt who is in charge of the relationship.

¤

Don't tell my wife.

¤

I was born an original and won't die a copy.

¤

I need you guys to stop writing me. As is noted in my profile, I'm heterosexual. If you keep asking me out I'm going to take down my picture.

¤

Into objectification, so if a Mistress is looking for a footstool, table or chair, I'm available.

¤

Got a big dick and a deep ass.

¤

I enjoy taking out a prospective partner and getting to know her properly in the vanilla world, before moving on to other things if the chemistry is there. If you enjoy quiet restaurants, comfortable chats, coffee shops, quiet pubs or clear starry nights, then we could be a match.

¤

Sexy, fit Scotsman loves raising his kilt for all sorts of kinky fun.

The End

Book #3- Fourteen Male/Female Anal Sex Stories

By Jennifer S.

Copyright (C) 2013

Fourteen Male - Female Anal Sex Scenes

1. My name is Erica. I'm a 114 lb pretty Mexican lady with straight black hair and full lips. My breast size is 32C. I was particularly proud of my firm very well proportioned ass that was perfect for playing with, and other things.

It was the morning on the 16th of December and as is the norm on weekdays I got on a very crowded subway to go to work. I was wearing a short black dress. I had black stockings on as well as black bra and panties. It was winter so I also wore a coat.

I was lucky enough to catch the express train even though it was packed. Nearly 15 minutes into the 45 minute ride I felt something brush against my ass as I stood holding onto the rail in the middle of the subway car. Then it happened again. Touching my ass is a huge turn on for me and I was still sleepy so I not only didn't get concerned about it but actually got turned on by it. Still I had forgotten about it when it happened a 3rd time. It was so crowded but I still tried turning around. I got a glimpse of a great looking guy looking down on me and standing right behind me. I knew it was him. He had a tie on and looked like an executive. He had a friendly but firm face. Then he leaned against my butt and now I was feeling his cock inside his pants. Suddenly the subway car went into a turn that forced my ass further into the cock. Suddenly I felt nothing and for the next 5 minutes I was horny as hell just thinking about what had just happened. If there was room I wanted to turn around and see what happened to him but what if he was gone and there was someone else there? What if I thought it was him but it was somebody else. I was very nervous but really turned on. Nothing like this had ever happened to me before.

Suddenly, a man whispered in my ear to stay still, not make a sound, and enjoy it. Soon I felt a hand on my so spankable ass slowly working its way down and under my skirt targeting my panties. Fingers went inside my panties and down the crack of my ass to my asshole. The next thing I knew my asshole was being taken by a lubricated finger, a long one too. The finger rammed my anus and stopped me right in my tracks. I was so turned on I didn't want to turn around or say anything that could interfere with this adventure, besides I love to have my asshole played with as much as I love to get taken in it.

My ass was being finger fucked by a pro for seemingly an eternity. He was very deliberate. He started out slowly then took me very fast then rested with slow thrusts and went back to fast pumping. Oh my gosh, what if I came right there in the subway car. It was so crowded and loud that if I was quiet nobody was likely to even notice, but suddenly it stopped and his delicious finger had partially been taken out of my ass. I stood there hoping for more, then, before I could turn around, my invader suddenly drove his finger in as far as it could go and left it there for the remainder of the ride, wiggling it regularly.

It was the most exciting subway ride I've ever had. While his finger rested inside of me I decided to try and cum. I closed my eyes and inconspicuously fucked his finger and sure enough had a nice, quiet orgasm as I held tight to the overhead rail so I wouldn't fall incase my knees buckled.

Then as we approached a stop, I felt his finger pull out of me. I wanted to turn around in case he wanted to get to know me better but was too shy to.

I arrived at the office and was horny the entire day. Later that evening I put my two vibrators to very good and lengthy use.

Every day I got on the subway at the same time looking for him. It was frustrating in a sense, but I really wondered what he was like and fantasized about having a date with him. Was he a great lover? Would he only want to take me in my ass?

I had given up on finding what in my mind I had somehow made into my dream man, when a week later I got on the subway to work and there he was. The subway wasn't as crowded then and even though I relished the thought of him finger fucking my ass again, it would be tougher to hid, besides there was an open seat next to him so I sat there. Would this be my only chance to get to know him better?

I couldn't ask him if he was the guy that played with my asshole like that as what if he wasn't. He could also be afraid to admit to it as he may be afraid he could get in trouble. He wasn't starting the conversation so I worked up the courage and asked him for the time. He was friendly and gave it to me and thankfully the conversation developed. We even agreed to meet for drinks later that day but my ass being finger fucked hadn't yet come up.

Well anyway I now live with him and yes that was him. Now he enjoys my asshole in many other ways and whenever he wants.

----

2. My boyfriend is the type who likes to fuck me in my ass, but still prefers to fuck my pussy, so I don't get it in the ass a real lot. I on the other hand love it in the ass. Therefore, I got pretty excited when Kevin called and said he was coming over to take me in the ass and I shouldn't have anything on, be on the bed waiting for him and already be well lubed. How nice, tonight I would have a little delicious pain and A LOT of pleasure.

30 minutes or so later he arrived. He had a key to my apartment so he walked right into the bedroom where I was eagerly waiting for him. His cloths were off in a flash and he sat down in front of me on the bed where I eagerly sucked on his cock. After 5 minutes of sucking, he lifted my head off of him and told me on to get on my hands and knees. He dried his hard cock off with a small towel so the condom would stick, put the condom on, lubed it, then entered my very ready ass.

"Does it hurt?" Kevin asked me, sliding another couple inches into me. I replied by shoving my ass back against him and taking the rest of his pulsing cock into my tight hole. His moans of pleasure told me that he was enjoying it too. He cautiously began pumping his cock in and out. I could tell he was concerned about hurting me. But as I'm the impatient type, I started pushing myself back into him, getting him to fuck me harder and faster. "Ooh yes" he said. "I'm going to cum in your tight little ass!"

That comment sent me over the edge, and I orgasmed long and hard. Just as I was finishing, I felt splashes of hot cum shooting deep inside my ass. It felt amazing, and it made me cum again.

Well this now has become a regular part of our playtime.

----

3. It was my boyfriend's birthday, and as well as a gift of a great shirt, I decided to give him another more personal present, my ass.

My name is Cindy and I'm a 29 year old brunette. 125 lbs, 5'3", 38 B boobs. Brad and I had been dating for a couple of months. He wanted to take me in my ass but I resisted it as I'd never experienced such a thing before. He had put toys in my ass when playing with me, and often when he was taking me doggie style, he would put a dildo in my lubricated ass which was attached to his body via a cord which was wrapped around his waist. Thus when he thrust into me, his pelvis pushed both his cock into my pussy as well as the dildo into my ass. It was great to be on my hands and knees with both of my holes being filled!

A few days ahead of time I told him on the phone about the special birthday present I was giving him, and I must admit that the anticipation was killing me. I couldn't wait. If I liked it I'd want us to do it a lot more often.

The night arrived and after a small birthday gathering at a bar, we returned for the main event.

Our clothes were off in a flash. I told him how I just couldn't wait for him to take me in my ass and how I had been thinking about it all week. He thought this would be a very memorable birthday present.

With my pussy at the edge of the bed, he ate it like it was dessert. With his birthday present in mind I gifted him with lots of pussy juice. He then told me to get further up on the bed and get on my elbows and knees. The moment was not far off. He then lubed my anus up pushing the lubrication deep and spending a lot of time finger fucking me. Little did he know how ready I was for this anal treat. He then sat against the head board and had me lay down on my stomach in front of him and make his cock hard with my mouth. I sucked away on his cock, sucking down his ooze as I made his cock harder and harder. I loved to feel a cock hardening in my mouth and clearly he was really enjoying himself too. Then suddenly he lifted my head off of his cock. The moment of truth had arrived.

He got behind me and oh my god I got entered! He started pumping my ass in a slow and deliberate motion. Like I envisioned all week, I loosened my anus as much as I could, and that seemed to make all the difference in the world. I figured I'd enjoy finally being taken in the ass and I did! Though I guess it helps to be so turned on.

Well that was a while back and being taken in the ass is a regular occurrence now. When we're having sex, Tom starts in my pussy and finishes in my ass!

----

4. The long and short of it is that I screwed up and accepted that my husband had the right to punish me. I would have preferred the usual spanking but he's done that so much with me over the years that mainly it just turns me on, so he thought of another punishment. I would have to wear a butt plug all day. He would put it on before we went to work and after we both got home he would take it out, at a time of his choosing. (We work at the same place in the garment district in Los Angeles. We had good jobs thanks to it being his family's business.)

He had put butt plugs in me before at different times for significant periods, such as when I was doing housework. Only on one other occasion however did I leave the house with a butt plug in me. It was once when I drove to the supermarket, with a stopover at the gas station for a fill-up, (of gas that is.)

I would have protested but I didn't know what other nasty punishment he would then do to me instead. (He can be very mischievous when it comes to punishing me.)

A very important part of this punishment was going to be which butt plug I would have to "wear". We had several. We had one he called the "spreader". It was 5 inches long and 1½ inches at its thickest point. There was one that was 6 inches long and an inch at its thickest. It looked like a penis and vibrated (mmmmm.) There is also the butt plug he called "ole reliable." It was 4 1/2" long and tapers to 1" at its widest. Then there were the anal beads. (As you can tell my asshole gets a lot of attention when it comes to sex.) He chose one of the anal beads.

Tomorrow would be Wednesday and that was determined to be the fateful day. Tomorrow came along and he picked my clothes out for me. I would be wearing a dark brown skirt, one of my stronger pairs of white panties (with an extra one in my purse just in case,) a white bra and a white button down blouse.

With just my bra on I put on my make-up then bent over a chair and waited as my husband came over, lubed me up well and inserted the anal bead toy well into my ass. Then using lots of white cloth first aid tape, he taped my asshole securely shut. After a quick spanking, we continued getting ready and I got in the car with him (often we take separate cars) but not today as he was having too much fun watching me fidget in my seat.

I would be allowed to lubricate my anus as much as I wanted throughout the day but I never did. If I was sitting I could pivot into a comfortable position. The bending down to sit could really get my attention. Getting up and walking was a different story and as the day progressed it made for some interesting moments.

Twice my husband called me down to the warehouse where he worked, to watch me walk. When no one was watching he had me bend over with my butt in front of him. Bending over was something I had to be very careful doing as the dildo stuck out a bit that way even though my muscles, the tape and my underwear mostly kept it in place. He had fun pushing it in even though it would quickly pop back towards him a bit. It also got me so turned on.

Still my anus felt raw after we got home and my husband finally took it out. But the sex that night was mind blowing!

----

5. I was on my hands and knees and Tom was kneeling behind me.

I found myself saying "Oh yes! I want more of you in me. I want you to finger fuck me like I've never been fucked before." I felt Tom slide yet another finger inside my pussy, then, without warning his lubricated, well manicured thumb entered my tight ass. I cried out and began bucking my hips against his hand. It hurt a bit but oh it felt so good.

"Oh god, fuck me hard." I felt Tom rocking his hand back and forth and up and down. First his fingers thrust into my pussy then his hand pulled out and up so his thumb could thrust even further into my ass. He pumped his finger in my ass all the while fucking my pussy with his other fingers. "Oh god yes! That feels so good!"

"What am I doing to you baby? Tell me."

"You're fucking my pussy with your fingers, and fucking my ass with your thumb."

Just then, Tom pulled out a finger in my pussy and also stuck it in my ass along with his thumb. Then he furiously fucked both my holes. "Now you've got two fingers in my ass. Yes, fuck me harder! Faster!"

I felt myself tightening up and Tom must have felt it also as he fucked my pussy and ass hard after slowing a bit for a rest. I exploded onto his hand and began bucking my hips against him. The orgasm I had was so intense, I heard myself ask him to stop, but I didn't mean it. I moaned and screamed, and suddenly I came again. In time Tom pulled his hand out of both my holes.

All I could do was lay there, completely exhausted. "Did you enjoy that baby?" Tom asked softly.

"Mmmmmmmmmmmmmmmmmmmmmmmmm" I replied as Tom kissed me tenderly before walking away.

----

6. My husband bought me a fucking machine for Christmas. It was an amazing surprise that I never expected. He goes on the road a significant amount so for that reason alone it would come in handy. Needless to say it got used often, which doesn't help our electricity bill!

One night though it was used on me for something unexpected, for punishment. I had forgotten to pay some bills which caused some problems to our credit rating. It was just a case of being forgetful and my husband wanted to nip that in the bud.

That night, at dinner, he informed me that my punishment tonight would be to be taken in the ass by the spanking machine, and only in the ass. We had tried anal sex before but I found it hurt but after screwing up our credit rating I found myself in no position to argue, and if anything felt I needed to be punished.

An hour or so after dinner, Jim told me to strip and wait for him next to the machine. I was nervous and even trembled from time to time. I knew Jim wanted to take me in my ass more often but it hurt, besides I exercised my pussy good and hard to make sure it was nice and tight for him.

Soon he came over and told me to "assume the position". I got on my elbows and knees at the usual spot and distance from the machine's arm that had the dildo at its end.

He didn't waste anytime either. He slowly slid the machine's dildo up into my ass. Even though it was thoroughly lubricated, it took a bit of time before it was finally stuffed all the way up my ass. I tried to ignore it and I hoped I would find it more comfortable later on. He then got up and went to the kitchen to get a drink.

When he came back I knew the time had come. There is a manual control lever on the fucking machine so one can manually make the machine's arm go back and forth; he activated that and my ass began to officially be taken.

He started slow and it made me moan. It did hurt some but starting slow like this was real helpful. I put my head down and loosen my asshole as much as I could.

What I really wanted to be able to do is cum from it. Also I knew that Jim at some point would sit in front of me and I'd be sucking on his cock while my ass was being taken.

"Keep your butt in place" he said. I didn't realize it but I was moving away some so less and less of the dildo was entering me. I quickly straighten out. Then Jim let the machine take over by turning it on.

The noise of the machine startled me but that ended up being a momentary concern. The fact is that fucking my ass was indirectly working my clit, even if my anus was the hole furthest from it.

The good news is that I was feeling okay and things would get better still as suddenly I heard the unmistakable humming of a vibrator next to me. Jim ran the vibrator along my pussy slowly then more quickly, and that would be the end of my fear of being taken anally!

"Oh yes, please, more…" Was that me that said that? Wow, it was. I actually was now humping the fucking machine and felt my first orgasm coming on. "Ohhhhhhhhhh." I put my head down and just hollered, "Oh god yes…more…" I came all over that vibrator and know my ass being fucked had a lot to do with it.

Jim then took away the vibrator and told me I had to cum from the ass fucking alone. I wanted so much to do that and knew I could. He got in front of me and sure enough I was sucking on his cock while my ass was being taken by the machine. It was amazing. He reached down and played with my boobs too. I now had two of my holes filled and my boobs being played with, but still no orgasm. 10 or so minutes later I was not only rewarded for all my sucking efforts with a mouth full of my husband's cum but I also came along with him as well!

Well I now often get taken by the fucking machine like that night, sometimes in my pussy, sometimes in my ass and sometimes in my pussy and then ass. Assuming my husband's home during that time I usually have his cock in my mouth, sucking the daylights out of it.

What a punishment that turned out to be!

----

7. After my boyfriend Joe spends some time fucking my pussy, it's time to take me in my ass. As part of foreplay he has already lubed my tight hole. He slowly puts his cock into my very tight asshole. It feels so tight going in but once it's in there, it feels incredible. Sometimes Joe fucks my ass really fast and sometimes he starts slow. I'll be moaning the whole time. I play with my clit and/or use a vibrator on my wet pussy. I fuck my pussy with my hand while Joe fucks my ass. His thrusts are very deep and very hard. We both love it so. Joe will spank me while taking me in my ass. It stings some but feels so good.

----

8. After watching TV in bed my husband and I decide to fuck, so we take off the rest of our clothes. After I suck on his cock to make it hard, my husband told me to get on my hands and knees. He then guides his very hard, thick cock into my dripping wet cunt. He thrusts deeper and deeper and it feels so incredible.

Soon his hands are all over my boobs and I turn my head and lean back so we can kiss deeply and passionately. He grabs my ass and starts to spank it, first lightly but the swats keep getting harder and harder and that feels great too. No words are usually spoken while we are lost in our hot, wild sex.

At some point my husband reaches for the lube and applies it to my tight hole, who's turn to be taken has come. He slowly glides his cock into my ass. I gasp a little at first from the delicious pain but he takes his time. At first he enters me slowly, but soon really starts to fuck my tight ass. He spanks my cheeks which make them a little sore but it feels great to be spanked while I'm being fucked in the ass. The thrusts are so deep and while he is fucking my sweet ass I am fucking my pussy with my fingers. I'm so wet that my pussy cums all over my fingers. I then take my fingers out of my wet cunt and let my husband taste them. He licks all the cum up and continues to fuck my ass harder and faster. Eventually he cums in my ass with a shout.

----

9. I love to ride Craig while Jon fucks me in the ass. I didn't like ass play until recently but I gave into their persistent requests as they told me they would be gentle and make me love it by the time we're finished. I start by straddling Craig and ride him with abandon. My pussy gets soaking wet as I ride him up and down. I then I push my ass up into the air and Jon lubes my tight ass and his cock. He slowly puts his first few inches into my ass. It feels different, but I'm so turned on that I don't feel it that much. He begins pushing more and more and now he is all the way in my tight ass. Oh my God, it feels amazing. Throughout all this I continue to fuck Craig. With two cocks now securely in me, I start to cum. "Oh god I'm going to cum" I scream. I cum as their cocks pound my pussy and ass.

In time we decide to switch. We would now stand up and I would get fucked like a sandwich. As I'm standing, Jon kind of holds me up and Craig does the same as it's now Craig's turn to fuck me in the ass. (Of course they use condoms and clean up before entering my pussy if previously been in my ass.) It was so different, bizarre, wild and dirty! As I'm cumming I tell them that I want to be their naughty slut who loves to suck and fuck.

Wow, I can feel their cocks bump against eachother from time to time through my flesh. Suddenly the testosterone really kicks in and they get into a competition to see who can fuck me in the hole they're in the hardest and fastest. We are like animals. What fun we are having. The sweat is pouring off our bodies and we are groaning and moaning like wild beasts. Gosh knows how many calories we burning! My pussy is dripping and all the friction felt great.

----

10. My husband spent over an hour last night playing with my anus. He wants to take me there but I think it's a sin so I say no, but he's so persistent so I agreed to let him play with it as long as he wants, as long as he doesn't take me there with his penis.

Well he now plays with my anus often using his fingers and sex toys. Last night was for the longest time by far.

Last night he sat on chair (we call it "the chair") in the middle of the room and told me to lay over his lap, like I would be if I was getting a spanking. We're both naked. Next to him on the right is small table. On it is what he'll use on me. It has the lube, sex toys (the use of which I don't think is a sin), towel to wipe me and/or himself off with and anything he is going to spank me with like paddles, a strap and sometimes even a hairbrush!

First though, after I was done cleaning up from dinner, we went into the bedroom and I gave him a long massage. As is normal we were both naked and while I straddled him, massaging him, he played with my breasts. I love it when he does that.

Finally it was time for me to use my mouth on his penis so he could have an orgasm. I laid down on my side and sucked away, feeling his cock get harder and harder in my mouth. It wouldn't be long before he filled my mouth with his seed.

We rested for a while then he told me it was time for us to go to the "chair". My husband just loves to play with my asshole. It took me a while to get used to it but now I really enjoy it.

I lay over his lap. He massaged my butt and legs then tells me to spread my legs. He then uses a vibrator on my vagina until I have an orgasm. It was so nice. But that was just the beginning. I then get a spanking with two of the paddles. During the spanking he'd use the vibrator on me again, often I can orgasm from just that but for some reason I couldn't last night. Then it was time for my anus to be played with, and it would be played with for a very long time!

After that we go back to the bedroom for intercourse.

----

11. My 34th birthday was one I would not forget. My fiancée promised me a special and unusual birthday and that is certainly what I got.

We've been together for almost two years. Our sexual interests have evolved a good deal. One of the things that's developed was our interest in anal sex. Now when we have sex, Jack starts in my pussy and finishes in my ass.

Ok, so after my birthday party, we were alone.

We kissed and cuddled on the couch for a while then Jack told me to go to the bedroom, strip, get on the bed and wait for my birthday surprise, which I did.

As he was about to enter the room he told me to close my eyes. I heard him enter and felt a bunch of stuff get dumped onto the bed in front of me. He said I could open my eyes and low and behold, sitting in front of me, was over a dozen brand new anal sex toys still in their wrappers! Jack told me that they all were going to get used on me tonight!

First I was scared and started to feel a tightness in my stomach, though also a throbbing between my legs. I bet I got wet then and there.

I looked the toys over. There were two anal trainer kits, couple of "lube shooters" to get the lube in all the way, 2 rump shakers, 6 butt plugs of various sizes, a vibrating anal probe, 3 sets of anal beads, all sorts of exotic lubes, a black throbbing anal balloon that gets inserted and inflated to stay securing in an ass, another expandable butt plug, 2 fingered butt plugs, an anal dilator kit and an oversized flesh colored butt plug that looked like trouble.

Well guess what we did nightly for some time! It was a blast, though sometimes I would need a night or two off for my asshole to regroup. After that night Jack would play with my ass with one or more of the anal toys, then we would make love.

Ladies what are you getting for your birthday?

----

12. You cover my eyes with a blindfold and tell me to bend over the back of the couch so my naked ass is in the air. I hear you moving behind me but don't know what to expect until I feel one of your lubricated fingers probing my tight little hole. You insert another wet finger which I can't help but start fucking. With your free hand you slap my ass hard and tell me to stay still. Then you remove your fingers and I feel another pressure against my hole. It's bigger than your fingers and I realize that it's a butt plug and from the feel of it one of the largest you have ever used on me. I want to pull away but know that wouldn't be right so I brace myself as you slide it in, which you do gently at first until the initial resistance of my muscles has passed, then you push hard so that the full length is in me. I moan again at this intrusion.

I hear a noise and realize that you inserted an inflatable butt plug and now you're inflating it. You inflate it past the point of comfort but I keep quiet. You then attach both of my hands together with handcuffs. You then tie ropes around each of my ankles which spread my legs good and wide, tying each ankle to opposite couch legs so my holes are on display for all to see. I am now immobile with my pussy and asshole sticking out very invitingly, even though my ass is full. Then you turn and leave the room. I am now alone and scared but I've been like this before so I start to feel a familiar tightness in my stomach and that wetness between my legs. I know that you will return and fuck me to your heart's content. Each thrust you make into me will also pound up against the inflated butt plug in me. While you're taking me you will reach down and play with my tits at will. I will cum so hard for you.

----

13. She said her name was Carla but who knows. She charged me $50 to fuck her in the ass. I never saw signs of STDs on her but again who knows. She would come over to my apartment, strip and jerk me off until I was hard. (Sometimes, unfortunately she would first go into the bathroom and snort cocaine before sex which was really uncool.) After she got me hard she would put a condom on me, lubed me up real good and get on her hands and knees, or elbows and knees. I didn't need to be particularly gentle in taking her in her ass and could slide right in and fuck hard within seconds. She loved it too. She would play with her clit with her hand and/or a vibrator. I'd spank her butt too as she'd start begging for that after a while.

She'd give me up to 20 minutes of ass fucking (I only fucked her in her pussy once but it was too loose and frankly I was pissed she even made me pay money for that.)

If I hadn't cum within 20 minutes, I'd pull out and she would lube my dick up even more and masturbate me to orgasm, which she was really good at actually.

Anyway, I heard she got busted for prostitution and hoped it wasn't anything worse. What sucked was I was afraid that the cops had gotten pictures of me with her or something, which fortunately they hadn't.

Anyway I really miss that tight ass and how much she enjoyed being fucked in it. I've fucked two ladies since but both wouldn't let me fuck their ass, which really sucks.

----

14. I'm a 36 year old white female that's been fucked in the ass many times. The first two times I was drunk which may be the best way to get acquainted with getting it in the ass.

I have a fuck buddy that loves fucking me in the ass. It was the first time for him and I think he hardly can believe his luck, not only am I a pretty no commitment fuck buddy but I love it up the ass too.

Well he did something the other night that blew me away. He called and told me to clean out my asshole really well (which I did before sex anyway.) He seemed really serious about it so I enemaed and soaped and did all the cleaning I could. Something was going on here as he was never like this. I also had to wonder if he wasn't freaking out in terms of thinking I was a dirty slut or something of that nature. That would be a hassle if I had to find another fuck buddy but doable as I went through dieting hell to get down to a size 6.

Anyway he came over to my place and we had the usual chit chat, watched American Idol and retired to my room when my nosey roommate came home.

Our clothes were off in a jiffy and wow did I ever have a treat, he ate out my asshole, as in with his mouth, and not for a minute or two but for 20-30 minutes!

He tongue fucked me several times throughout it all, often he played with my clit during all this.

I had never had this done to me and after I got over the surprise, I realized how excited I was. Fortunately I had 2 different vibrators within arm's reach and I put them to quick use on and in my pussy. My orgasms were amazing.

Girls if you're into anal sex you've got to experience this. Warning to the guys, tongue fucking an asshole for a long time can really make your tongue sore!

The End